STEVEN CHEN

Sauna & Cryotherapy

Step by Step Guide to Boost Cognitive Performance, Reduce Stress, Enhance Mental Resilience, and Promote Longevity

Contents

Introduction

In today's fast-paced world, the demands on our minds and bodies are greater than ever. Balancing work, family, and personal growth often leaves us feeling drained and stressed. But what if there were simple, science-backed practices that could not only restore your energy but also enhance your mental clarity, resilience, and overall well-being? Welcome to the transformative worlds of sauna and cryotherapy.

This book is your condensed guide to harnessing the power of thermal and cold therapy without sifting through 100's of pages of research. Rooted in ancient traditions and supported by modern science, these therapies offer profound benefits for both mind and body. Whether you're looking to boost cognitive performance, reduce chronic stress, build mental resilience, or promote longevity, sauna and cryotherapy provide a practical, effective path to achieving these goals.

In these pages, you'll find a step-by-step approach to integrating these therapies into your life. We'll explore the science behind their benefits, including how they influence your brain, hormones, and immune system. You'll also learn how to tailor these practices to suit your unique needs and lifestyle, ensuring you can safely and effectively reap their rewards.

From seasoned athletes to busy professionals, from wellness enthusiasts to those new to self-care, sauna and cryotherapy are tools that anyone can use to unlock their full potential. As you embark on this journey, remember: the path to a sharper mind, a calmer spirit, and a longer, healthier life begins with small, consistent steps.

Let's take the first one together.

1

Chapter 1: What Are Sauna and Cryotherapy?

For centuries, humans have harnessed the power of temperature extremes to promote healing, relaxation, and vitality. From the steaming, wood-paneled rooms of Finnish saunas to the icy chambers of modern cryotherapy, these practices tap into the body's innate ability to adapt, recover, and thrive. But what exactly are sauna and cryotherapy, and why have they gained such a devoted following?

Sauna: Heat Therapy with Ancient Roots

The sauna is one of the oldest and most celebrated forms of heat therapy, dating back thousands of years. Originating in Finland, the sauna was traditionally a wooden hut or room heated by a stove or fire, where people would gather to cleanse their bodies and relax their minds. Today, saunas come in many forms, including traditional wood-burning models, infrared saunas that use light waves to heat the body directly, and electric saunas that provide convenience and consistency.

At its core, the sauna works by exposing the body to intense heat, typically ranging from 150 to 195°F (65 to 90°C). This heat triggers a cascade of physiological responses: your heart rate increases, blood vessels dilate, and sweat glands work overtime. The result? Improved circulation, detoxification, and a profound sense of relaxation.

Modern science has added new dimensions to the sauna's appeal, revealing benefits like enhanced cardiovascular health, reduced inflammation, and improved mental clarity. For many, the sauna is not just a place to unwind—it's a tool for optimizing physical and mental performance.

Cryotherapy: The Science of Cold Exposure

In stark contrast to the soothing heat of the sauna is the invigorating chill of cryotherapy. This practice, derived from the Greek words *kryos* (cold) and *therapeia* (heal), involves exposing the body to extremely low temperatures for short durations. Cryotherapy can take various forms, from localized ice packs and cold water immersions to whole-body cryotherapy (WBC) chambers cooled to temperatures as low as -220°F (-140°C).

Unlike heat therapy, cryotherapy rapidly cools the skin, prompting a survival response that sends blood rushing to your core to protect vital organs. Once the session ends, freshly oxygenated and nutrient-rich blood flows back to the extremities, promoting recovery and reducing inflammation.

Cryotherapy is particularly popular among athletes for its ability to accelerate muscle recovery and reduce soreness. But its benefits extend far beyond the athletic world, offering potential relief for chronic pain, improved mental focus, and even anti-aging effects.

A Synergy of Extremes

While sauna and cryotherapy may seem like polar opposites, they share a common goal: to stimulate the body's natural adaptive processes. Heat and cold therapy both trigger stress responses that, when applied thoughtfully, can strengthen the body and mind. Many enthusiasts combine these therapies in contrast sessions, moving between the intense heat of a sauna and the icy chill of cryotherapy to maximize their benefits.

This dual approach is rooted in hormesis—a principle where exposure to manageable stressors helps the body adapt and become stronger. By leveraging this concept, sauna and cryotherapy offer a unique, science-backed method for enhancing resilience, promoting recovery, and unlocking peak performance.

In the chapters that follow, we'll dive deeper into the science behind these therapies and explore step-by-step guides to incorporating them into your life. Whether you're seeking relaxation, cognitive enhancement, or a path to longevity, sauna and cryotherapy provide powerful tools to help you achieve your goals.

2

Chapter 2: The Benefits of Sauna Use

Saunas have been celebrated for centuries as a space for relaxation, rejuvenation, and social connection. But beyond their soothing warmth lies a treasure trove of health benefits that extend far beyond mere comfort. Modern science has revealed that regular sauna use can profoundly improve physical, mental, and emotional well-being. In this chapter, we explore the powerful benefits of sauna therapy and how it can help you unlock your full potential.

1. Enhanced Cardiovascular Health

One of the most well-documented benefits of sauna use is its positive effect on cardiovascular health. The intense heat causes your heart rate to increase, mimicking the effects of moderate exercise. Blood vessels dilate, through a process known as vasodilation, improving circulation and delivering oxygen-rich blood throughout your body. Studies have shown that regular sauna sessions can:

- Lower blood pressure by improving arterial flexibility.
- Reduce the risk of cardiovascular diseases, including heart attacks and strokes.
- Promote heart health by enhancing the function of the endothelium (the lining of blood vessels).

Regular sauna use has been shown to improve cardiovascular health by enhancing blood circulation, which can help reduce the risk of heart disease. A study published in the *Journal of the American College of Cardiology* found that frequent sauna bathing is associated with a lower risk of sudden cardiac death, coronary artery disease, and overall cardiovascular mortality.

For individuals unable to engage in traditional physical exercise, sauna use offers a gentle yet effective alternative for supporting cardiovascular fitness.

2. Stress Reduction and Mental Clarity

The sauna's calming environment provides a perfect escape from the pressures of daily life. Heat exposure triggers the release of endorphins, your body's natural feel-good chemicals, leading to a sense of relaxation and well-being. The heat activates the parasympathetic nervous system (the "rest and digest" system), which counteracts the fight-or-flight response and promotes a state of relaxation. This results in reduced levels of the stress hormone cortisol, which, when chronically elevated, can impair cognitive function.

Regular sauna use has been shown to:

- Reduce levels of cortisol, the stress hormone, promoting a calmer state of mind.

- Enhance mental clarity and focus, thanks to improved blood flow to the brain.
- Support emotional resilience, making it easier to handle stressors with grace.

A sauna session can serve as a mental reset, offering a break to recharge and refocus in the midst of a hectic schedule. The feeling of calmness and mental rejuvenation following a sauna session is why many people use it as a tool to unwind after a stressful day or to promote mental resilience.

3. Detoxification and Skin Health

Sweating is one of your body's natural mechanisms for detoxification. In the sauna, the heat stimulates intense sweating, helping to eliminate toxins such as heavy metals, environmental pollutants, and metabolic waste. A study conducted by the University of Finland found that sauna bathing increased the excretion of lead, mercury, and other toxic metals, suggesting that sauna use may be an effective strategy for supporting the body's natural detoxification processes.While the kidneys and liver are the primary detox organs, sweating in the sauna provides an additional means of eliminating waste, leading to a deeper level of detoxification.

This detoxification process can lead to:

- Improved skin health, as sweat helps to cleanse pores and promote a healthy glow.
- Enhanced lymphatic function, supporting your immune system's ability to remove waste.
- A stronger defense against inflammation, as toxins are

flushed out of your system.

For those seeking a natural way to support their body's detox pathways, the sauna is a powerful ally.

4. Boosted Cognitive Performance

Heat exposure in the sauna triggers the production of brain-derived neurotrophic factor (BDNF), a protein that supports the growth and maintenance of neurons. This process can lead to:

- Improved memory and learning abilities, as BDNF strengthens neural connections.
- A reduced risk of neurodegenerative diseases, such as Alzheimer's and Parkinson's.
- Enhanced mood and creativity, thanks to better brain function and blood flow.

Many sauna users report feeling sharper and more creative after a session, making it an excellent tool for boosting cognitive performance.

5. Pain Relief and Muscle Recovery

Sauna therapy is a favorite among athletes and active individuals for its ability to soothe sore muscles and accelerate recovery. The heat increases blood flow to muscles, delivering nutrients and oxygen to promote healing. Benefits include:

- Reduced muscle soreness after intense physical activity.
- Relief from chronic pain, including conditions like arthritis

and fibromyalgia.
- Improved flexibility and joint mobility, as heat relaxes tight muscles and connective tissue.

Whether you're recovering from a workout or dealing with chronic pain, sauna sessions can be a natural way to find relief.

6. Immune System Support

Regular sauna use has been linked to a stronger immune system. The heat mimics a mild fever, stimulating the production of white blood cells and activating immune defenses. This can result in:

- Increased resistance to colds and infections, especially during flu season.
- Faster recovery from illness, as immune function is heightened.

By making the sauna a part of your routine, you can bolster your body's natural defenses against illness.

7. Longevity and Overall Well-being

Perhaps most exciting is the growing body of evidence linking sauna use to increased lifespan. A large-scale study conducted in Finland found that individuals who used a sauna four to seven times per week had a 40% lower risk of dying from cardiovascular disease and a 50% lower risk of dying from other causes compared to those who used a sauna only once a week. This correlation between sauna use and increased longevity is thought to result from the cumulative effects of improved heart health, stress reduction, and cellular protection.

Sauna use has also been shown to improve the quality and depth of sleep, primarily by promoting relaxation and reducing tension in the body. The rise in body temperature followed by a cooling-off period after leaving the sauna triggers the body's natural sleep mechanisms, making it easier to fall asleep and stay asleep. Better sleep leads to improved memory consolidation, enhanced focus, and faster cognitive recovery, which are essential for performance well-being.

Studies have found that individuals who use saunas regularly experience:

- Lower mortality rates, particularly from cardiovascular and respiratory diseases.
- Improved quality of life, as both physical and mental health are enhanced.
- Slowed aging, thanks to reduced inflammation and oxidative stress.
- Improved quality of sleep.

By promoting cellular repair and reducing chronic stressors, sauna therapy serves as a powerful tool for supporting longevity.

The science behind sauna use reveals a fascinating array of benefits for the body and mind. From boosting cardiovascular health and promoting detoxification to enhancing cognitive performance and supporting longevity, sauna bathing is a powerful wellness practice. As more research uncovers the long-term effects of heat exposure on the body and brain, it's clear that sauna use is not just a relaxing activity but a scientifically supported tool for optimizing health and well-being.

In the following chapters, we will explore how to safely incorporate sauna use into your routine and how to combine it with cryotherapy for even greater benefits. By understanding the science behind these therapies, you can fully harness their potential to improve your physical, mental, and emotional resilience.

3

Chapter 3: Step-by-Step Guide to Getting Started with Sauna Use

Sauna therapy is a simple yet profoundly effective practice for improving physical and mental health. If you're new to saunas, you might feel uncertain about how to begin, what to expect, or how to maximize the benefits. This chapter provides a step-by-step guide to help you confidently incorporate sauna use into your wellness routine.

Step 1: Choose the Right Sauna

There are various types of saunas available, each with unique features and benefits. Here's a quick overview to help you decide:

1. Traditional Saunas

- Uses heated stones or a stove to create dry heat.
- Temperature: 150–195°F (65–90°C).
- Offers an intense, classic sauna experience.

2. Infrared Saunas

- Uses infrared light to heat your body directly, rather than heating the air.
- Temperature: 120–140°F (49–60°C).
- Ideal for a gentler heat that penetrates deeply into muscles.

3. Steam Saunas

- Produces moist heat by generating steam.
- Temperature: 110–120°F (43–49°C).
- Great for respiratory health and skin hydration.

Visit local spas or wellness centers to try different types, or invest in a home sauna for added convenience.

Step 2: Prepare for Your Sauna Session

Proper preparation ensures you can fully enjoy and benefit from your sauna experience.

1. Hydrate

- Drink plenty of water before your session to replenish fluids lost through sweating.
- Avoid alcohol or caffeine, as they can dehydrate you further.

2. Choose the Right Time

- Saunas are most effective when used after exercise or at the end of the day to relax.

- Avoid heavy meals or fasting before your session, as it may cause nausea.

3. Gather Essentials

- Bring a towel to sit on and another to dry off.
- Consider wearing a light cotton towel or going nude, depending on the sauna rules and your comfort level.
- Optional: Bring water, sandals, moisturizer, lotion, essential oils, or a timer.

Step 3: Start Slowly and Gradually Build Tolerance

When using a sauna for the first time, it's essential to ease into the experience.

1. Begin with Short Sessions

- Start with 5–10 minutes to allow your body to adapt to the heat.
- Gradually increase your time over a few sessions, aiming for 15–30 minutes per visit.

2. Listen to Your Body

- Sauna use should feel relaxing, and maybe uncomfortable in the beginning, but not life threatening.
- If you feel dizzy, nauseous, or lightheaded, exit the sauna immediately and cool down.

3. Experiment with Temperature

- Start at a lower temperature and increase as you become more comfortable.
- Infrared saunas tend to feel less intense than traditional saunas at the same temperature.

Step 4: Enhance Your Sauna Experience

To maximize the benefits and enjoyment, consider these tips:

1. Use Aromatherapy

- Add a few drops of essential oils like eucalyptus or lavender to the sauna rocks or a nearby bowl of water for a calming or invigorating scent. Practice Deep Breathing
- Focus on slow, steady breaths through your nose to relax your body and mind.
- This also helps improve respiratory health in steam or traditional saunas.

2. Incorporate Meditation or Music

- Use your time in the sauna for mindfulness or light meditation.
- Some saunas come with Bluetooth capabilities for calming music or nature sounds.

3. Alternate with Cool-Down Periods

- After your session, step out and cool down for a few minutes with a cold shower, pool plunge, or fresh air.
- Repeat this cycle if you're doing multiple rounds.

Step 5: After Your Sauna Session

How you recover and hydrate after your session is just as important as the session itself.

1. Rehydrate

- Drink plenty of water or electrolyte-rich fluids to replace lost minerals.
- Coconut water or an electrolyte drink can be especially helpful.

2. Cool Down Gradually

- Allow your body to return to its normal temperature naturally.
- Avoid jumping into cold water immediately after if you're new to sauna use.

3. Moisturize Your Skin

- After sweating, cleanse and moisturize your skin to maintain its hydration and health.

Step 6: Create a Sauna Routine

Consistency is key to reaping the full benefits of sauna therapy.

1. Set a Schedule

- Start with 2–3 sessions per week, adjusting based on your goals and how your body responds.
- As you build tolerance, you can increase the frequency if desired.

2. Track Your Progress

- Keep a journal of how you feel after each session to identify the benefits and adjust your routine.
- Pay attention to changes in stress levels, energy, and sleep quality.

3. Pair Sauna with Other Wellness Practices

- Combine sauna use with exercise, mindfulness, or cold therapy (cryotherapy) to enhance overall well-being.

Step 7: Stay Safe

While saunas are generally safe, it's important to follow these precautions:

1. Know Your Limits

- Avoid prolonged sessions or excessive heat, especially if you're new to saunas.

- If you have medical conditions, consult your doctor before starting sauna therapy.

2. Avoid Alcohol

- Alcohol consumption before or after a sauna session can increase the risk of dehydration and overheating.

3. Stay Aware

- Avoid using a sauna alone, especially if you're a beginner. Having someone nearby ensures safety in case of dizziness or overheating.

By following this step-by-step guide, you can ease into sauna therapy with confidence and build a sustainable practice that aligns with your health goals. In the next chapter, we'll delve into the science of cryotherapy and how to integrate cold exposure for complementary benefits to sauna use.

4

Chapter 4: The Benefits of Cryotherapy Use

Cryotherapy, or cold therapy, is a practice that dates back centuries, evolving from simple ice baths to advanced cryo chambers that expose the body to extreme cold in a controlled environment. Although its icy embrace might seem daunting at first, cryotherapy offers a host of powerful health benefits for both mind and body. In this chapter, we explore the science-backed advantages of cryotherapy and how it can elevate your wellness journey.

1. Accelerated Muscle Recovery and Reduced Inflammation

Cryotherapy is widely celebrated for its ability to soothe sore muscles and reduce inflammation, making it a favorite among athletes and active individuals. Cold exposure constricts blood vessels, decreasing inflammation and swelling. As the body warms back up post-treatment, oxygenated blood rushes to the affected areas, promoting healing and recovery.

Key Benefits:

- Faster recovery from intense workouts or physical activity.
- Relief from conditions like tendonitis, arthritis, and other inflammatory issues.
- Improved mobility and reduced joint stiffness.

For athletes or anyone with a physically demanding lifestyle, cryotherapy is a game-changer in speeding up recovery times and reducing downtime.

2. Boosted Immune System Function

Cold exposure stimulates the production of white blood cells, which are essential for a robust immune system. Regular cryotherapy sessions can enhance the body's natural defenses, helping you stay healthier year-round.

Key Benefits:

- Increased resistance to common illnesses like colds and flu.
- Strengthened immune response to combat infections and diseases.

By challenging the body with short bursts of cold, cryotherapy triggers an adaptive response that fortifies overall immunity.

3. Enhanced Cognitive Performance and Mental Clarity

Cold therapy has proven to improve brain health and cognitive function. Cryotherapy stimulates the release of norepinephrine, a neurotransmitter that improves focus, attention, and mood. Additionally, the rush of oxygen-rich blood post-session delivers vital nutrients to the brain, enhancing mental clarity.

Key Benefits:

- Improved concentration, memory, and mental sharpness.
- Reduced brain fog and enhanced productivity.
- Support for mental resilience under stress.

Many users report feeling invigorated and mentally recharged after cryotherapy, making it an excellent tool for peak cognitive performance.

4. Stress Relief and Mood Enhancement

Cryotherapy isn't just about physical recovery—it also profoundly impacts emotional well-being. Exposure to extreme cold triggers the release of endorphins and other feel-good chemicals like serotonin and dopamine, creating a natural mood boost.

Key Benefits:

- Reduced symptoms of anxiety and depression.
- Enhanced emotional balance and resilience.
- A calm, uplifted mood following each session.

For those struggling with the pressures of daily life, cryotherapy offers a quick and effective way to reset the mind and elevate mood.

5. Pain Management

Cryotherapy's ability to reduce inflammation and numb nerve endings makes it a powerful tool for managing chronic pain conditions. It's particularly beneficial for individuals with musculoskeletal issues or persistent pain that interferes with daily life.

Key Benefits:

- Alleviation of pain from conditions like fibromyalgia, arthritis, and migraines.
- Improved quality of life for those living with chronic discomfort.
- A drug-free alternative for pain relief.

Whether you're recovering from an injury or managing a long-term condition, cryotherapy can provide significant and lasting relief.

6. Improved Skin Health and Anti-Aging Effects

Cryotherapy has gained popularity in the beauty and skincare world for its rejuvenating effects on the skin. The cold constricts blood vessels and reduces puffiness, while increased circulation post-treatment helps repair skin cells and boost collagen production.

Key Benefits:

- Firmer, more youthful skin due to improved elasticity and

collagen synthesis.
- Reduced appearance of wrinkles, redness, and puffiness.
- A brighter, healthier complexion.

Regular cryotherapy sessions can support your skin's natural healing processes, making it an excellent addition to an anti-aging routine.

7. Metabolism Boost and Weight Management

Cold exposure activates brown adipose tissue (BAT), a type of fat that burns energy to generate heat. This process, known as thermogenesis, can increase your metabolic rate and support weight management.

Key Benefits:

- Increased calorie burn even after the session ends.
- Support for fat loss through activation of brown fat.
- Enhanced metabolic health and energy balance.

While cryotherapy isn't a magic weight-loss solution, it can complement a healthy diet and exercise program to improve metabolic efficiency.

8. Hormesis and Longevity

Cryotherapy is a prime example of hormesis—a process where small doses of stress stimulate the body to adapt and become stronger. Over time, this adaptive response can contribute to increased resilience, improved cellular repair, and overall longevity.

Key Benefits:

- Reduced oxidative stress and inflammation, key factors in aging.
- Enhanced cellular repair and mitochondrial function.
- Greater overall vitality and a longer, healthier life.

By incorporating cryotherapy into your routine, you're not only improving how you feel today but also investing in your future health and longevity.

Making Cryotherapy Work for You

The benefits of cryotherapy are vast, but they're most effective when used consistently and thoughtfully. Whether you're seeking relief from pain, a boost in mental clarity, or support for long-term wellness, cryotherapy offers a versatile and powerful tool to help you reach your goals.

In the next chapter, we'll dive into the practical side of cryotherapy, providing a step-by-step guide to getting started and safely incorporating it into your lifestyle. From preparing for your first session to developing a sustainable routine, we'll cover everything you need to know to make the most of this transformative practice.

5

Chapter 5: Step-by-Step Guide to Cryotherapy Use

Cryotherapy, or cold therapy, has been gaining popularity as a powerful tool for enhancing physical and mental health. Whether used for reducing inflammation, improving recovery after exercise, or boosting cognitive performance, the therapeutic effects of cryotherapy are supported by a growing body of scientific research. This chapter will guide you through the step-by-step process of using cryotherapy effectively, ensuring that you harness its full potential to improve your health, reduce stress, and enhance mental resilience.

What is Cryotherapy?

Cryotherapy involves exposing the body to extremely cold temperatures for a short period to trigger a range of beneficial physiological responses. The most common form of cryotherapy is whole-body cryotherapy (WBC), where the body is exposed to temperatures as low as -200°F (-129°C) for 2–3 minutes.

Localized cryotherapy, which targets specific areas of the body (such as muscles or joints), involves similar cold treatments but applied to only one part of the body. Alternative forms of cold therapy such as cold showers and cold plunges can also be utilized to ease the body into extreme temperatures.

Cryotherapy stimulates the body's natural healing processes, reduces inflammation, improves circulation, and supports mental clarity and resilience. With that background, let's dive into a step-by-step guide on how to safely and effectively use cryotherapy.

Step 1: Choose the Right Cryotherapy Option

There are two main types of cryotherapy: **whole-body cryotherapy (WBC)** and **localized cryotherapy**. Alternative cold therapies include: **ice plunge** and **cold shower**.

- **Whole-body cryotherapy (WBC):** This is done in a chamber or cryo-sauna that cools the air to extremely low temperatures. The entire body is exposed to the cold, usually for 2–3 minutes. WBC is typically used for overall wellness, recovery, and boosting cognitive performance.
- **Localized cryotherapy:** Involves applying cold to specific areas of the body, such as knees, shoulders, or back, using a device that delivers cold air or a liquid nitrogen stream. Local cryotherapy is beneficial for reducing pain, inflammation, and promoting targeted recovery.
- **Ice Plunge:** This can be done in a bathtub or cold plunge

tub easily accessible on Amazon. Fill the tub with cold water and ice, then immerse your whole body into the tub from anywhere between 1-5 minutes. While the cold plunge won't reach as low temperatures as WBC, it is a useful DIY alternative that can be cost-effective if you're on a budget.

- **Cold Shower:** This can be done so long as you have access to a shower. Turn on the showerhead and leave the valve at the coldest temperature available. Shower as you normally would with hot water and reap the benefits. This is the most convenient method to tap into cold therapy without spending an extra dime.

Choosing the right cryotherapy option depends on your goals. For those looking to push their peak potential, whole-body cryotherapy remains the gold standard. For targeted pain relief or recovery from injury, localized cryotherapy is ideal. For general wellness and cognitive enhancement, the cold plunge is the preferred method. For the most cost-effective and convenient method, the cold shower is readily available at home.

Step 2: Prepare for Your Cryotherapy Session

Preparation is key to ensuring a safe and effective cryotherapy experience. Follow these steps to prepare your body and mind:

1. **Hydrate:** Proper hydration is essential before any cryotherapy session. Drink plenty of water to ensure your body can handle the cold and facilitate optimal circulation.
2. **Avoid heavy meals and alcohol:** It's best not to eat a

large meal or drink alcohol right before your cryotherapy session. These can affect your circulation and overall comfort during the treatment.

3. **Wear appropriate clothing:** For WBC, you'll typically be asked to wear minimal clothing (such as socks, gloves, and underwear) to protect sensitive areas of your body from extreme cold. Avoid wearing jewelry or makeup as these can interfere with the cold's contact with your skin.

4. **Mental preparation:** Cryotherapy can be intense, especially during the first few minutes. Mentally prepare yourself by focusing on your breath and reminding yourself of the benefits you'll experience. It's helpful to stay calm and focused throughout the session.

Step 3: Undergo the Cryotherapy Session

Once you're prepared, the cryotherapy session begins. Here's what you can expect during your treatment:

Whole-Body Cryotherapy (WBC)

1. **Enter the Cryo Chamber or Sauna:** For WBC, you'll step into the cryotherapy chamber or cryo-sauna, where the air temperature will drop significantly. The chamber typically has an open design, and you'll stand inside while the cold air surrounds your body. The temperature in the chamber will be set to between -200°F (-129°C) and -300°F (-184°C).

2. **Stay Inside for 2–3 Minutes:** The session typically lasts 2–3 minutes. During this time, your body will experience

an intense cold shock that causes blood vessels to constrict and your body to work hard to preserve core temperature.

3. **Monitor Your Comfort:** Cryotherapy can feel intense, but most people report that the cold is bearable after the first few seconds. The temperature is very low, but you'll remain comfortable as your body adapts. If you begin to feel lightheaded or uncomfortable, inform the technician immediately.

4. **Exit the Cryotherapy Chamber:** After the session ends, you'll exit the chamber and begin the rewarming process. Your body will naturally start to warm up as your circulation returns to normal, and you'll begin to feel invigorated.

Localized Cryotherapy

1. **Target Area Application:** If you're using localized cryotherapy, a technician will use a hand-held device to direct cold air or nitrogen to the targeted area of your body, such as your knee, shoulder, or back. This process usually takes about 10–15 minutes per area.

2. **Cold Exposure:** As the cold air is applied, the targeted area will feel an intense but tolerable chill. Similar to whole-body cryotherapy, the cold induces vasoconstriction in the area, reducing inflammation and promoting healing.

3. **End of Session:** Once the treatment is complete, the targeted area may feel numb or tingly as circulation returns to normal. The recovery is typically quick and often involves gentle movements to restore flexibility and mobility to the treated area.

Ice Plunge

1. **Set up the Tub:** You can use a home bathtub or purchase an ice plunge tub online. Next, fill half the tub with cool water and fill another quarter of the tub with ice. Make sure not to fill the tub to the top or you may overflow the tub once you enter. Wait about 3 minutes for the ice to settle.

2. **Immerse Yourself:** Once the tub is ready, slowly lower your whole body into the tub with only your head above water. For beginners, try 30 seconds to 1 minute for your first session. Then gradually increase the time, aiming for 3–5 minutes per session.

3. **End of Session:** Once you're done, use the handrails or sides of the tub to slowly stand and exit the tub. Dry off with a towel as you allow your body temperature to reach homeostasis before continuing on with your day.

Cold Shower

1. **Enter the Shower:** Turn on the shower head and set the valve to the coolest comfortable temperature. Adjust the temperature slowly to build tolerance, until you've reached the coldest temperature available. This method offers similar healing properties, but allows individuals to go at their own pace.

2. **Cold Exposure:** As the cold water runs, adjust the temperature slowly to build tolerance, until you've reached the coldest temperature available. This method offers similar healing properties, but allows individuals to go at their own pace.

3. **End of Session:** Once you're done, slowly exit the shower. Dry off with a towel as you allow your body temperature to reach homeostasis.

Step 4: Post-Cryotherapy Care

After your cryotherapy session, it's important to follow a few steps to maximize the benefits and support your body's recovery:

1. **Warm Up Gradually:** In the case of whole-body cryotherapy, your body will begin to warm up naturally after exiting the chamber. However, if you still feel chilled, dress in warm clothes or take a warm shower to encourage your body to return to a comfortable temperature.
2. **Hydrate Again:** Rehydrate after your session to help replenish fluids lost during the treatment and support the body's recovery. Hydration will help keep your circulation strong and your muscles flexible.
3. **Avoid Intense Physical Activity Immediately:** After cryotherapy, it's a good idea to avoid strenuous exercise for a few hours. This gives your body time to recover fully and allow the anti-inflammatory effects to take hold. However, light stretching or walking can be helpful to keep your blood circulating.
4. **Observe for Side Effects:** While most people tolerate cryotherapy well, some may experience mild redness or irritation at the site of treatment. These effects should subside within an hour or so. If you experience anything more severe, contact a healthcare provider.

Step 5: Integrating Cryotherapy into Your Routine

For optimal results, cryotherapy should be integrated into a regular wellness routine. Here's how you can incorporate it effectively:

1. **Frequency:** Depending on your goals, aim to undergo cryotherapy 2–3 times per week for best results. For specific issues like injury recovery or chronic pain, you may benefit from more frequent sessions.
2. **Combine with Other Wellness Practices:** Cryotherapy works well in conjunction with other wellness practices, such as sauna use, exercise, and meditation. You might find that combining sauna sessions with cryotherapy enhances both mental clarity and physical recovery.
3. **Track Your Progress:** Keep track of how you feel before and after each cryotherapy session. This can help you monitor improvements in cognitive function, mood, and physical performance over time.

Cryotherapy is a powerful tool for boosting cognitive performance, reducing stress, enhancing mental resilience, and promoting overall wellness. By following this step-by-step guide, you can ensure that you are using cryotherapy safely and effectively. Whether you are a professional athlete, a busy executive, or simply someone seeking to improve your health, cryotherapy has the potential to support your body's natural healing processes, enhance recovery, and improve both physical and mental well-being.

6

Chapter 6: Warnings, Safety, and Proper Use

While sauna and cryotherapy are powerful tools for enhancing health and well-being, they involve exposing the body to extreme conditions. As with any wellness practice, safety and proper usage are paramount to avoid potential risks. In this chapter, we outline important precautions, contraindications, and best practices to ensure you can safely reap the benefits of these therapies.

General Safety Guidelines

Whether you are using a sauna or cryotherapy, the following general guidelines apply:

1. Consult with a Healthcare Provider

- If you have any medical conditions, are pregnant, or are taking medications, consult your doctor before starting sauna or cryotherapy.

- People with cardiovascular issues, respiratory conditions, or neurological disorders should exercise caution.

2. Listen to Your Body

- Never push through discomfort, dizziness, or nausea. These are signs that you need to stop immediately.
- If you feel faint or unwell during or after a session, seek medical attention.

3. Stay Hydrated

- Both therapies can lead to significant fluid loss through sweating (in saunas) or physiological responses to cold (in cryotherapy). Drink plenty of water before and after each session.

4. Limit Session Duration

- Overexposure can lead to adverse effects such as dehydration, heat exhaustion, or frostbite. Always adhere to recommended time limits.

Sauna Safety Tips

1. Temperature and Duration

- Start with lower temperatures and shorter durations, especially if you're new to sauna use.
- Avoid exceeding 20–30 minutes per session unless you are

highly experienced.

2. Avoid Alcohol and Heavy Meals

- Alcohol dehydrates the body and impairs judgment, increasing the risk of overheating.
- Heavy meals before a session can cause discomfort or nausea.

3. Supervise Use

- Never use a sauna alone, particularly if you're a beginner or have health concerns.
- Children and older adults should use saunas only under supervision and with adjusted temperatures and durations.

4. Cool Down Gradually

- After a session, allow your body to return to a normal temperature slowly. Abrupt cooling (such as a plunge into icy water) can cause shock to your system.

5. Avoid Overuse

- Daily sauna use is not necessary for optimal benefits and can lead to dehydration or mineral imbalances. Start with 2–4 sessions per week.

Cryotherapy Safety Tips

1. Duration and Temperature

- Whole-body cryotherapy (WBC) sessions should last no more than 2–3 minutes.
- Ensure the cryo-chamber temperature is set correctly, usually between -200°F to -300°F (-130°C to -150°C).

2. Protect Vulnerable Areas

- Always wear protective gear, including gloves, socks, and ear coverings, to prevent frostbite.
- Avoid direct contact with metal jewelry or wet clothing, which can cause burns.

3. Avoid Cryotherapy with Open Wounds

- Do not use cryotherapy if you have open sores, wounds, or skin conditions like eczema, as the cold can worsen these issues.

4. Monitor for Cold Intolerance

- If you experience tingling, numbness, or pain during a session, exit the cryo-chamber immediately.
- Individuals with Raynaud's disease or sensitivity to cold should approach cryotherapy with caution.

5. Pregnancy and Medical Conditions

- Pregnant individuals should avoid cryotherapy due to potential risks to fetal health.

- Conditions such as severe hypertension, heart arrhythmias, or a history of frostbite may also avoid use.

Understanding Risk Factors

While sauna and cryotherapy are generally safe for healthy individuals, certain conditions can increase risks.

Risk Factors for Sauna Use:

- Severe cardiovascular disease or uncontrolled hypertension.
- Fever or acute illnesses, such as infections.
- Epilepsy or heat-sensitive neurological disorders.
- Pregnancy (consult with a healthcare provider).

Risk Factors for Cryotherapy Use:

- Severe cold intolerance or Raynaud's phenomenon.
- History of frostbite or cold-induced conditions.
- Poor circulation, such as peripheral artery disease.
- Uncontrolled high blood pressure or recent heart attacks.

If you have any of these conditions, seek medical advice before proceeding.

Tips for Maximizing Benefits Safely

1. Start Slow and Build Tolerance

- Gradually increase the intensity of your sessions as your

body adapts.

- For saunas, this means starting with lower temperatures and shorter durations. For cryotherapy, begin with shorter exposures to cold.

2. Combine Therapies Mindfully

- If using sauna and cryotherapy together, alternate between sessions with adequate rest periods.
- Avoid jumping straight from one extreme to the other without allowing your body to normalize.

3. Monitor Progress and Adjust

- Keep track of how your body responds to each session.
- If you notice any negative effects, reduce session frequency or duration and consult a professional.

4. Stay Consistent, Not Excessive

- Both therapies are most effective when used regularly but not excessively. Stick to a schedule that allows for recovery and balance.

Emergency Situations and How to Respond

In rare cases, sauna or cryotherapy may cause adverse reactions. Here's what to do:

1. Overheating (Sauna)

- Symptoms: Dizziness, headache, or rapid heartbeat.
- Response: Exit the sauna immediately, hydrate, and rest in a cool environment.

2. Cold-Induced Issues (Cryotherapy)

- Symptoms: Numbness, frostbite, or difficulty breathing.
- Response: Exit the chamber, warm the affected areas gently (avoid hot water), and seek medical attention if necessary.

3. Fainting or Loss of Consciousness

- In both cases, remove the individual from the environment, lay them flat, and call for emergency assistance.

By understanding these precautions and following best practices, you can safely enjoy the transformative benefits of sauna and cryotherapy. In the next chapter, we'll explore how to create a balanced wellness routine that integrates these therapies into your lifestyle effectively and sustainably.

7

Chapter 7: Post-Sauna and Cryotherapy Checklist

The benefits of sauna and cryotherapy don't end when you step out of the heat or cold. What you do immediately after your session plays a critical role in amplifying the effects of these therapies. A proper post-session routine helps your body recover, rehydrate, and maximize the physical and mental benefits. This chapter provides a comprehensive checklist to guide you through the essential steps to take after each session.

1. Hydrate Thoroughly

Both sauna and cryotherapy can leave your body dehydrated— saunas through sweating and cryotherapy through increased metabolic activity. Replenishing fluids is the first step to recovery.

Checklist:

- Drink at least 12–16 ounces of water immediately after your session. Listen to your body if you need more or less.
- Consider electrolyte-enhanced drinks or coconut water to restore lost minerals.
- Avoid alcohol and caffeine, which can exacerbate dehydration.

2. Nourish Your Body

After a session, your body is in an optimal state to absorb nutrients. Eating the right foods can enhance recovery and energy levels.

Checklist:

- Choose light, nutrient-rich snacks like fresh fruits, nuts, or a protein smoothie.
- Incorporate anti-inflammatory foods such as berries, leafy greens, or omega-3-rich salmon.
- Avoid heavy, greasy meals that may cause sluggishness.

3. Cool Down or Warm Up Gradually

After a sauna session, your body needs time to cool down naturally. Similarly, after cryotherapy, gradual warming is key to avoiding shock to your system.

Checklist for Sauna:

- Rest in a cooler but comfortable environment for 10–15 minutes.
- Consider a lukewarm or cold shower to close your pores and remove sweat.
- Avoid jumping into an ice bath immediately unless you are experienced with contrast therapy.

Checklist for Cryotherapy:

- Warm up gently with light movements or a warm blanket if needed.
- Avoid hot showers or heating pads immediately after a session, as they can interfere with the benefits of cold exposure.

4. Stretch or Move Lightly

Post-session, your muscles are relaxed and more pliable, making it an ideal time for light stretching or gentle movement.

Checklist:

- Perform dynamic stretches to increase flexibility and relieve tension.
- Practice light yoga or slow walking to maintain blood flow and prevent stiffness.
- Avoid intense workouts immediately after, as your body needs time to recover.

5. Support Skin Health

Both therapies impact your skin, so taking care of it post-session can enhance their rejuvenating effects.

Checklist:

- Rinse your skin with water to remove toxins and sweat.
- Use a gentle, hydrating moisturizer to replenish moisture, especially after cryotherapy.
- Avoid harsh soaps or exfoliants immediately post-session to prevent irritation.

6. Rest and Recover

Your body needs time to process and integrate the effects of the session. Rest is a crucial part of the recovery process.

Checklist:

- Schedule downtime after your session to relax and recover fully.
- Consider a short nap or quiet time to allow your nervous system to reset.
- Avoid overloading your schedule with intense physical or mental tasks right after.

7. Reflect and Track Progress

Keeping a record of your post-session experience helps you tailor your routine and identify patterns in how your body responds to sauna and cryotherapy.

Checklist:

- Note how you feel physically and mentally (e.g., energy levels, mood, and muscle recovery).
- Track metrics such as heart rate variability, sleep quality, or pain relief if applicable.
- Adjust the frequency, duration, or intensity of sessions based on your observations.

8. Integrate Mindfulness

Both sauna and cryotherapy create an ideal state for mindfulness and mental clarity. Use this time to deepen your mind-body connection.

Checklist:

- Practice gratitude or journal about your experience and how you feel.
- Incorporate breathing exercises or meditation to extend the calming effects.
- Set intentions for your next session, focusing on specific goals like relaxation, recovery, or performance enhancement.

9. Plan Your Next Session

Consistency is key to maximizing the long-term benefits of sauna and cryotherapy. Having a plan ensures you stay on track with your wellness goals.

Checklist:

- Schedule your next session based on your recovery needs and routine.
- Balance sauna and cryotherapy with other wellness practices like exercise, nutrition, and sleep.
- Monitor how you feel in the days following to decide the ideal frequency for your body.

Your post-session routine is just as important as the session itself. By following this checklist, you can create a seamless recovery process that enhances the immediate and long-term benefits of sauna and cryotherapy.

8

Final Thoughts

Congratulations on taking the journey through the transformative practices of sauna and cryotherapy. By now, you've gained a deeper understanding of how these therapies can unlock your potential for physical vitality, mental clarity, and overall well-being.

From the ancient traditions of sauna bathing to the cutting-edge innovations of cryotherapy, both approaches have proven to be more than fleeting wellness trends. They are time-tested and scientifically supported methods for boosting cognitive performance, reducing stress, enhancing mental resilience, and promoting longevity.

Embracing Balance in Your Wellness Journey

Wellness is not about quick fixes or rigid routines—it's about creating a sustainable balance that aligns with your goals and lifestyle. Sauna and cryotherapy are powerful tools, but their true magic lies in how they integrate with your broader wellness habits. When paired with mindful nutrition, regular exercise, quality sleep, and self-care practices, these therapies can amplify your efforts and elevate your health to new heights.

As you continue your journey, remember that consistency and mindfulness are key. Listen to your body, adapt your routine as needed, and enjoy the process of becoming your healthiest, most vibrant self.

In Summary

This book has equipped you with practical steps to:

- Understand the science and history behind sauna and cryotherapy.
- Harness the benefits of these therapies safely and effectively.
- Customize your routine to suit your unique needs and goals.
- Avoid potential risks through proper precautions and informed decisions.

The real value of this knowledge comes from putting it into practice. Whether you're using these therapies to recover from workouts, find mental clarity, or support longevity, each session is an opportunity to invest in yourself.

A Call to Action

Your health is your greatest asset, and the power to enhance it is in your hands. Take what you've learned here and make sauna and cryotherapy a meaningful part of your routine. Share your experiences with others and inspire them to explore these therapies for themselves.

In a world where stress and busyness often dominate, prioritizing your wellness isn't just a gift to yourself—it's a statement of self-respect and a commitment to living your best life.

Thank you for joining me on this journey. May the lessons in this book guide you toward a healthier, happier, and more resilient future. Here's to your well-being and longevity!

If you found this book helpful, I'd be very appreciative if you left a favorable review for the book on Amazon!

Warm (and cool) regards,

Anna B. Rivers

Resources

Doidge, N. (2007). *The brain that changes itself: Stories of personal triumph from the frontiers of brain science.* Viking.

Fletcher, N., et al. (2019). The role of heat stress and cold exposure in regulating stress resilience. *Frontiers in Psychology, 10,* 1516. https://doi.org/10.3389/fpsyg.2019.01516

Freedman, M. (2011). *How to live forever: The enduring power of connecting the generations.* PublicAffairs.

Greitens, E. (2015). *Resilience: Hard-won wisdom for living a better life.* Houghton Mifflin Harcourt.

Hohenauer, E., et al. (2018). The effects of cryotherapy on physical recovery and athletic performance. *International Journal of Sports Medicine, 39*(12), 937-944. https://doi.org/10.1055/a-0677-8759

Laukkanen, J. A., & Kunutsor, S. K. (2018). Effects of sauna bathing on cardiovascular and cerebrovascular health. *European Journal of Preventive Cardiology, 25*(4), 441–447. https://doi.org/10.1177/2047487318775972

Longo, V. (2018). *The longevity diet: Discover the new science behind stem cell activation and regeneration to slow aging, fight disease, and optimize weight.* Penguin Books.

Lubkowska, A., et al. (2015). Whole-body cryotherapy: A review of the benefits and risks. *Therapeutic Advances in Musculoskeletal Disease, 7*(5), 219–227. https://doi.org/10.1177/1759720X15600144

Mayo Clinic. (2021). Whole-body cryotherapy: What to know before trying it. *Mayo Clinic.* Retrieved from https://www.mayoclinic.org

National Center for Biotechnology Information (NCBI). (2020). The science behind sauna and cryotherapy: Exploring the benefits. *NCBI.* Retrieved from https://www.ncbi.nlm.nih.gov

Southwick, S. M., & Charney, D. S. (2012). Resilience in the face of adversity: The science of stress and the secrets of coping. *Current Psychiatry Reports, 14*(5), 534–540. https://doi.org/10.1007/s11920-012-0327-8

Tugade, M. M., & Fredrickson, B. L. (2004). Psychological resilience and stress management in healthy adults: A review. *Journal of Social and Clinical Psychology, 23*(6), 807–848. https://doi.org/10.1521/jscp.23.6.807.54888

WebMD. (2020). Cryotherapy: What you should know before trying it. *WebMD.* Retrieved from https://www.webmd.com

Zaccaria, M., et al. (2021). Sauna bathing and systemic inflammation: A review of current research. *Journal of Science and Medicine in Sport, 24*(9), 868-875. https://doi.org/10.1016/j.jsams.2020.11.013

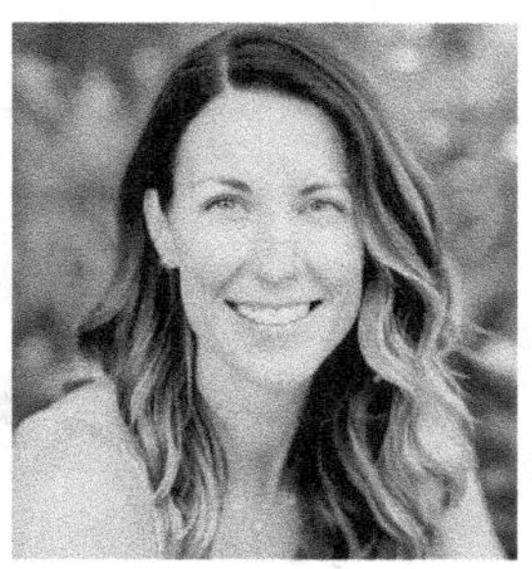

About the Author

Anna B. Rivers is a passionate advocate for holistic wellness and a lifelong learner in the pursuit of optimizing mind and body performance. With a deep interest in science-based approaches to health, Anna has dedicated years to exploring practices that enhance cognitive function, mental resilience, and overall longevity.

Her journey began with a personal quest to overcome stress and achieve balance in a demanding world. This led her to discover the transformative benefits of sauna and cryotherapy. Combining her research skills with hands-on experience, Anna has mastered these techniques and developed practical strategies to help others incorporate them into their lives.

As a writer, Anna's mission is to empower readers with tools and knowledge that are both accessible and practical. She brings together ancient traditions and cutting-edge science, presenting them in a way that is easy to understand and apply.

When she's not writing, Anna enjoys experimenting with wellness trends, hiking in nature, and practicing mindfulness. Through her work, she hopes to inspire others to embrace small, intentional changes that lead to big, lasting results.

In *Sauna & Cryotherapy: Step by Step Guide to Boost Cognitive Performance, Reduce Stress, Enhance Mental Resilience, and Promote Longevity*, Anna distills her expertise into an actionable guide, inviting readers to unlock their potential and thrive in both mind and body.